Study Guide to Accompany

Foundations of Maternal & Pediatric Nursing
Third Edition

Study Guide to Accompany

Foundations of Maternal & Pediatric Nursing

Third Edition

Lois White, RN, PhD,

Gena Duncan, MSEd, MSN,

Wendy Baumle, MSN

Prepared by
Cheryl Pratt, RN, MA, CNAA-BC
Regional Director of Nursing
School of Nursing
Rasmussen College

Previous edition prepared by
Kathleen Peck Schaefer, RNC, MSN, MEd
Brandy Coward, BSN

DELMAR
CENGAGE Learning

Australia • Brazil • Japan • Korea • Mexico • Singapore • Spain • United Kingdom • United States

Foundations of Maternal & Pediatric Nursing Study Guide, Third Edition

By Lois White, RN, PhD, Gena Duncan, MSEd, MSN, and Wendy Baumle, MSN

Vice President, Career and Professional Editorial: Dave Garza

Director of Learning Solutions: Matt Kane

Executive Editor: Steven Helba

Managing Editor: Marah Bellegarde

Senior Product Manager: Juliet Steiner

Editorial Assistant: Meghan E. Orvis

Vice President, Career and Professional Marketing: Jennifer Ann Baker

Executive Marketing Manager: Wendy Mapstone

Senior Marketing Manager: Michele McTighe

Marketing Coordinator: Scott Chrysler

Production Director: Carolyn Miller

Production Manager: Andrew Crouth

Senior Content Project Manager: James Zayicek

Senior Art Director: Jack Pendleton

For product information and technology assistance, contact us at **Professional & Career Group Customer Support, 1-800-648-7450**

For permission to use material from this text or product, submit all requests online at **cengage.com/permissions**. Further permissions questions can be e-mailed to **permissionrequest@cengage.com**.

Library of Congress Control Number: 2010920488
ISBN-13: 978-1-4283-1786-4
ISBN-10: 1-4283-1786-4

Delmar
5 Maxwell Drive
Clifton Park, NY 12065-2919
USA

Cengage Learning products are represented in Canada by Nelson Education, Ltd.

For your lifelong learning solutions, visit **delmar.cengage.com**
Visit our corporate website at **cengage.com**.

NOTICE TO THE READER

Publisher does not warrant or guarantee any of the products described herein or perform any independent analysis in connection with any of the product information contained herein. Publisher does not assume, and expressly disclaims, any obligation to obtain and include information other than that provided to it by the manufacturer. The reader is expressly warned to consider and adopt all safety precautions that might be indicated by the activities described herein and to avoid all potential hazards. By following the instructions contained herein, the reader willingly assumes all risks in connection with such instructions. The publisher makes no representations or warranties of any kind, including but not limited to, the warranties of fitness for particular purpose or merchantability, nor are any such representations implied with respect to the material set forth herein, and the publisher takes no responsibility with respect to such material. The publisher shall not be liable for any special, consequential, or exemplary damages resulting, in whole or part, from the readers' use of, or reliance upon, this material.

Printed in the United States of America
1 2 3 4 5 6 7 14 13 12 11 10

Contents

Preface

This Study Guide is designed to accompany *Foundations of Maternal & Pediatric Nursing*, Third Edition, by Lois White, Gena Duncan, and Wendy Baumle. Each of the eight chapters in this guide was created to facilitate student learning and refine student skills. By using this guide at home and in the clinical setting, you will work with important concepts and begin to apply them to real-life situations.

To facilitate your learning, each chapter in this guide includes the following components:

- *Key Terms Review*: a matching exercise designed to enhance your understanding of new terms presented in the text.
- *Abbreviation Review*: exercise to test your knowlege of abbreviations, acronyms, and symbols used in the text.
- *Exercises and Activities*: short scenarios with related questions to test your understanding and application of concepts.
- *Self-Assessment Questions*: multiple-choice questions that draw on the key ideas in the chapter and prepare you to succeed in your examinations.

Prenatal Care

Key Terms

Match the following terms with their correct definitions.

___ 1. Abortion

___ 2. Age of viability

___ 3. Amenorrhea

___ 4. Amnion

___ 5. Anticipatory guidance

___ 6. Ballottement

___ 7. Blastocyst

___ 8. Braxton-Hicks contractions

___ 9. Chadwick's sign

___10. Chloasma

___11. Chorion

___12. Coitus

___13. Colostrum

___14. Copulation

___15. Cotyledon

___16. Couvade

___17. Decidua

a. Delivery after 24 weeks' gestation but before 38 weeks (full term).

b. False pregnancy.

c. Sexual act that delivers sperm to the cervix by ejaculation of the erect penis.

d. Gestational age at which a fetus could live outside the uterus, generally considered to be 24 weeks.

e. Descriptor for a pregnancy between 38 and 42 weeks' gestation.

f. Rebounding of the floating fetus when pushed upward though the vagina or abdomen.

g. Fetal vessel connecting the pulmonary trunk to the aorta.

h. Structure that connects the fetus to the placenta.

i. Absence of menses.

j. Loss of pregnancy before the age of viability, usually considered to be 24 weeks.

k. White, creamy substance covering the fetus's body.

l. Information, teaching, and guidance given to a client in anticipation of an expected event.

m. Darkening of the skin of the forehead and around the eyes; also called "mask of pregnancy."

n. Fecal material stored in the fetal intestines.

o. Practice of eating substances not considered edible and that have no nutritive value such as laundry starch, dirt, clay, and freezer frost.

p. Delivery after 42 weeks' gestation.

q. Fertilized ovum.

____18. Ductus arteriosus

____19. Ductus venosus

____20. Fertilization

____21. Foramen ovale

____22. Fundus

____23. Funic souffle

____24. Goodell's sign

____25. GP/TPAL

____26. Gravida

____27. Hegar's sign

____28. Implantation

____29. Lanugo

____30. Leopold's maneuvers

____31. Linea nigra

____32. Meconium

____33. Morula

____34. Multigravida

____35. Multipara

____36. Nesting

____37. Nulligrava

____38. Nullipara

r. Condition of being pregnant for the first time.

s. Lowering of blood pressure in a pregnant woman when lying supine due to compression of the vena cava by the enlarged, heavy uterus.

t. Inner fetal membrane originating in the blastocyst.

u. Sexual act that delivers sperm to the cervix by ejaculation of the erect penis.

v. Flap opening in the atrial septum that allows only right to left movement of blood.

w. Condition of having delivered once after 24 weeks' gestation.

x. Thick substance surrounding and protecting the vessels of the umbilical cord.

y. Care of a woman during pregnancy, before labor.

z. Outer fetal membrane formed from the trophoblast.

aa. Irregular, painless uterine contractions felt by the pregnant woman toward the end of pregnancy.

bb. Mental and physical preparation for childbirth; synonymous with Lamaze.

cc. Purplish blue color of the cervix and vagina noted at about week 8 of pregnancy.

dd. Development of physical symptoms by the expectant father such as fatigue, depression, headache, backache, and nausea.

ee. Pregnancy, regardless of duration, including present pregnancy.

ff. Descriptor for when the mother feels the fetus move, about 16 to 20 weeks' gestation.

gg. The mammalian conceptus in the postmorula stage.

hh. Hemodilution caused by the increased maternal blood volume.

ii. Membranous vascular organ connecting the fetus to the mother, which produces hormones to sustain a pregnancy, supplies the fetus with oxygen and food, and transports waste products out of the fetal system.

jj. Reddish streaks frequently found on the abdomen, thighs, buttocks, and breasts; also called stretch marks.

kk. Series of specific palpations of the pregnant uterus to determine fetal position and presentation.

ll. Top of the uterus.

___39. Para

mm. Dark line on the abdomen from umbilicus to symphysis during pregnancy.

___40. Physiologic anemia of pregnancy

nn. Agent such as radiation, drugs, viruses, and other micro-organisms capable of causing abnormal fetal development.

___41. Pica

oo. Sound of blood pulsating through the uterus and placenta.

___42. Placenta

pp. Condition of being pregnant two or more times.

___43. Polyhydramnios

qq. Branch of the umbilical vein that enters the inferior vena cava.

___44. Postterm

rr. Condition of having delivered twice or more after 24 weeks' gestation.

___45. Prenatal care

ss. Embedding of a fertilized egg into the uterine lining.

___46. Preterm

tt. Antibody-rich yellow fluid secreted by the breasts during the last trimester of pregnancy and first 2 to 3 days after birth; gradually changes to milk.

___47. Primigravida

uu. Fine hair covering the fetus's body.

___48. Primipara

vv. Softening of the cervix noted about week 8 of pregnancy.

___49. Pseudocyesis

ww. Condition of never having been pregnant.

___50. Psychoprophylaxis

xx. Softening of the uterine isthmus about week 6 of pregnancy.

___51. Quickening

yy. Gravida, para/term, preterm, abortions, living.

___52. Striae gravidarum

zz. Condition of having delivered (given birth) after 24 weeks' gestation, regardless of whether infant is born alive or dead or number of infants born.

___53. Supine hypotensive syndrome

aaa. Subdivision on the maternal side of the placenta.

___54. Teratogen

bbb. Union of an ovum and a sperm.

___55. Term

ccc. Sound of blood pulsating through the umbilical cord; rate the same as the fetal heartbeat.

___56. Umbilical cord

ddd. Surge of energy late in pregnancy when the pregnant woman organizes and cleans the house.

___57. Uterine souffle

eee. Condition of never having delivered an infant after 24 weeks' gestation.

___58. Vernix caseosa

fff. The endometrium after implantation of the trophoblast.

___59. Wharton's jelly

ggg. A solid mass of cells formed by cleavage of a zygote.

___60. Zygote

hhh. Excessive amniotic fluid.

Abbreviation Review

Write the meaning or definition of the following abbreviations, acronyms, and symbols.

1. ASPO _____

2. AWHONN _____

3. BOW _____

4. BPD _____

5. C-H _____

6. C-R _____

7. DES _____

8. EDB _____

9. EDD _____

10. GP/TPAL _____

11. GFR _____

12. hCG _____

13. Hgb F _____

14. hPL _____

15. ICEA _____

16. LMP _____

17. NAACOG _____

18. OTC _____

19. PBI _____

Exercises and Activities

1. What is the importance of prenatal care for the woman and her baby?

   _____

   _____

   _____

   _____

2. List several factors that can affect the development of the fetus.

   (1) _____   (5) _____

   (2) _____   (6) _____

   (3) _____   (7) _____

   (4) _____   (8) _____

3. Your client is a 23-year-old with insulin-dependent diabetes who is hoping to become pregnant within the next year. Why is it important for her to begin preconception care now?

   _____

   _____

   _____

4. Describe the physiological changes and symptoms that occur with pregnancy in the following systems.

   Cardiovascular: _____

   _____

Respiratory: _____

_____

Musculoskeletal: _____

_____

Gastrointestinal: _____

_____

Urinary: _____

_____

5. Draw a line under each of the "probable" signs of pregnancy, and draw a circle around those that are "positive" signs.

Amenorrhea	Abdominal enlargement	Chadwick's sign
Funic souffle	Breast tenderness	Braxton-Hicks contractions
Fatigue	Goodell's sign	Fetus visualization
Quickening	Uterine enlargement	Uterine souffle
Ballottement	Chloasma	Hegar's sign
Positive pregnancy test	Morning sickness	Linea nigra
Fetal heartbeat	Fetal movement by examiner	

6. List four developmental tasks of pregnancy.

   (1) _____

   (2) _____

   (3) _____

   (4) _____

7. How does the father or support person prepare for the birth of the baby?

   _____

   _____

8. What causes each of these common discomforts? Identify two or more interventions that can help to relieve each one.

	Cause	Interventions
Nausea/vomiting		
Constipation		
Ankle edema		
Dyspnea		
Leg cramps		
Dizziness/fainting		

9. F.M. is a 29-year-old mother of two children, ages 3 and 7, and is now 34 weeks pregnant. F.M. tells you that she wants to do everything she can to prepare her children for the birth of their new baby brother or sister. What suggestions can you give her?

_____

_____

_____

10. The nurse asks you to review the warning signs for hypertension/preeclampsia with F.M. before she leaves today. What information will you include?

_____

_____

11. Convert each of the following to the abbreviated form (G_P_/T_P_A_L_) for these clients.
    (1) _____   Second pregnancy, one child at home who was born at 38 weeks
    (2) _____   First pregnancy (now at 22 weeks)
    (3) _____   Pregnant for the third time; the first pregnancy ended in a miscarriage at 11 weeks; the second ended with a full-term birth; one living child at home
    (4) _____   Nulligravida
    (5) _____   Second pregnancy with twins; first pregnancy resulted in twins born at 34 weeks, who are doing well

12. Using Naegele's rule, calculate the EDB for each of the following:

    LMP July 9   EDB _____
    LMP December 22   EDB _____
    LMP February 1   EDB _____
    LMP May 15   EDB _____

13. S.B. is a 23-year-old child-care worker who is pregnant for the second time. She tells you that her first child, a 3-year-old boy, was born prematurely at 34 weeks but is doing well now. S.B. says that she was so young when she had her first baby that she didn't feel ready. She had no prenatal care until late in the pregnancy. S.B. would have preferred to become pregnant next year rather than now. However, this time she really wants to take care of herself and have a full-term, healthy baby.

    a. You write on the prenatal assessment form that S.B. is G__P__/T__P__A__L__.
    The date of her LMP was June 12, so you note that her EDB is _____.

    b. S.B. appears to be completing the first developmental task of pregnancy because:

    _____

    _____

    c. S.B. is about nine weeks pregnant now. When you ask about any discomforts that she may be experiencing, she tells you that she is having some heartburn and mood swings. You advise her to:

    _____

    _____

d. Besides a thorough health history, what else will the first visit include?

_____

_____

e. S.B. has a few questions for you. Can you help?

"How soon can you hear the baby's heartbeat?" _____

"How big is the baby right now?" _____

"When will I feel the baby move?" _____

"How often do I have to come to the clinic?" _____

"I want to know if it's a boy or a girl. Can I get an ultrasound to find out?" _____

f. S.B. returns for one of her follow-up prenatal visits when she is 28 weeks pregnant.

What would you expect for a fundal height measurement at this time? _____

What is the approximate weight gain you would expect by this time? _____

What other tests will probably be done at this visit?

_____

_____

g. You mention the childbirth classes your hospital offers. S.B. says, "I've been through this once already, so I don't see how going to classes would really help me. Nothing helps labor, anyway." What would you tell her about the benefits of attending a prepared childbirth class?

_____

_____

_____

_____

_____

_____

14. Write in the possible cause for each warning sign in pregnancy.

Warning Sign	Possible Cause
Vaginal bleeding (any), bloody show	
Sudden gush of fluid from the vagina	
Persistent vomiting	
Sever continuous headache	
Swelling of face, hands, legs, feet when rising in the morning	
Visual disturbances: blurring, double vision, flashes of light, spots before eyes	
Dizziness	
Fever over 100°F	
Pain in abdomen or cramping	
Epigastric pain	
Irritating vaginal discharge	
Dysuria	
Oliguria	
Noticeable reduction or absence of fetal movement	

Self-Assessment Questions

Circle the letter that corresponds to the best answer.

1. The nurse measuring the fundal height of a client who is 20 weeks pregnant finds it at the level of her umbilicus. The nurse determines that this
   a. is a normal finding.
   b. is greater than expected.
   c. indicates oligohydramnios.
   d. requires an immediate ultrasound.

2. You review lab work on your client, who is 32 weeks pregnant. You note that she has a hematocrit of 34%. This is most likely caused by
   a. iron deficiency anemia.
   b. poor dietary intake of protein.
   c. placental transport of blood to the fetus.
   d. hemodilution from an increase in plasma.

3. When the client complains about the Braxton-Hicks contractions she is experiencing, the nurse explains that their purpose is to
   a. soften and dilate the cervix.
   b. help her to practice breathing techniques.
   c. help with uterine and placental circulation.
   d. improve the abdominal muscle tone for delivery.

4. A client has gone into labor at 23 weeks of gestation. The nurse understands that this is below the age of viability for the infant because
   a. there is an absent suck/swallow reflex.
   b. alveoli are insufficient for air exchange.
   c. the infant has fetal hemoglobin present.
   d. the fetus has passed meconium in utero.

5. A client in the prenatal clinic is scheduled to have the following tests during her pregnancy. Which of these would be used to screen for possible birth defects?
   a. Venereal Disease Research Laboratory
   b. Rubella titer
   c. Coomb's test
   d. Alpha-fetoprotein

6. A nurse is reviewing data for her client, a 37-year-old primigravida who is now at 35 weeks' gestation. Her blood pressure today is 150/85, and she is complaining of mild edema in her legs. You determine that according to her usual blood pressure of 120/68, this is
   a. high and needs to be reported.
   b. a typical increase in the last month of pregnancy.
   c. abnormal only if the client also has edema in her hands and face.
   d. a result of a later maternal age in an otherwise normal pregnancy.

7. Fathers who smoke and mothers who do not
   a. have lower-birth-weight infants.
   b. have infants who are unaffected.
   c. have large-for-gestational age infants.
   d. have normal-weight infants.

8. The trophoblast secretes _____ during the early pregnancy.
   a. estrogen
   b. progesterone
   c. hPL
   d. hCG

9. The fetal stage of development from the beginning of week 3 through week 8 is called
   a. germinal stage.
   b. embryonic stage.
   c. fetal stage.
   d. cephalo stage.

10. At what week of fetal development is lanugo only on the shoulders and upper back?
    a. Week 28
    b. Week 32
    c. Week 36
    d. Week 40

Complications of Pregnancy

Chapter 2

Key Terms

Match the following terms with their correct definitions.

____ 1. Abortion

____ 2. Abruptio placenta

____ 3. Amniocentesis

____ 4. Biophysical profile

____ 5. Early deceleration

____ 6. Eclampsia

____ 7. Ectopic pregnancy

____ 8. Euglycemia

____ 9. HELLP syndrome

____10. Hydatidiform mole

____11. Hydramnios

____12. Hyperemesis gravidarum

____13. Incompetent cervix

____14. Kernicterus

a. Pregnancy in which the fertilized ovum is implanted outside the uterine cavity.

b. Reduction in fetal heart rate that begins after the uterus has begun contraction and increases to the baseline level after the uterine contraction has ceased.

c. Assessment of five variables: fetal breathing movement, fetal movements of body or limbs, fetal tone (flexion/extension of extremities), amniotic fluid volume, and reactive NST.

d. Termination of a pregnancy before viability of the fetus, usually 24 weeks.

e. Withdrawal of amniotic fluid to obtain a sample for specimen examination.

f. Abnormality of the placenta wherein the chorionic villi become fluid-filled, grapelike clusters; the trophoblastic tissue proliferates; and there is no viable fetus.

g. Deficiency in the amount of amniotic fluid.

h. Reduction in fetal heart rate that begins early with the contraction and virtually mirrors the uterine contraction.

i. Excessive fetal growth characterized by a fetus weighing more than 4,000 g (8.8 lb).

j. Reduction in fetal heart rate that has no relationship to contractions of the uterus.

k. Normal blood glucose level.

l. Premature separation, from the wall of the uterus, of normally implanted placenta.

m. Convulsion occurring in pregnancy-induced hypertension.

n. Pregnancy-induced hypertension with liver damage characterized by hemolysis, elevated liver enzymes, and low platelet count.

___15. Late deceleration

___16. Macrosomia

___17. Miscarriage

___18. Modified biophysical profile

___19. Oligohydramnios

___20. Placenta previa

___21. Preeclampsia

___22. Tocolysis

___23. Variable deceleration

o. Spontaneous abortion.

p. Excessive vomiting during pregnancy.

q. Condition in which the placenta forms over or very near the internal cervicalos.

r. Excess amount of amniotic fluid.

s. Descriptor for when the cervix begins to dilate, usually during the second trimester.

t. Phase of pregnancy-induced hypertension prior to convulsions.

u. Severe neurological damage resulting from a high level of bilirubin (jaundice).

v. Process of stopping labor with medications.

w. Assessment of the NST and amniotic fluid volume to determine fetal wellness.

Abbreviation Review

Write the meaning or definition of the following abbreviations, acronyms, and symbols.

1. CMV _____

2. CST _____

3. CVS _____

4. D&C _____

5. DIC _____

6. EDB _____

7. EFM _____

8. FAST _____

9. FBPP _____

10. FHR _____

11. FHT _____

12. GDM _____

13. hCG _____

14. HELLP _____

15. hPL _____

16. HSV-2 _____

17. IUGR _____

18. L/S _____

19. $MgSO_4$ _____

20. MSAFP _____

21. NST _____

22. PG _____

23. PIH _____

24. PKU _____

25. RhoGam _____

26. SGA _____

27. TORCH _____

28. VST _____

Exercises and Activities

1. What role does fetal assessment play during pregnancy?

   _____

   _____

2. If a pregnancy is determined to be high-risk, what monitoring may be used to assess fetal well-being?

   _____

   _____

3. List several abnormal conditions that can be detected with ultrasound.

   (1) _____   (4) _____

   (2) _____   (5) _____

   (3) _____   (6) _____

4. Describe a "normal" finding for a nonstress test.

   _____

   _____

5. Describe a "normal" finding for a contraction stress test.

   _____

   _____

   _____

6. Identify the variables that are assessed with a biophysical profile.

   (1) _____

   (2) _____

   (3) _____

   (4) _____

   (5) _____

7. What information is obtained with each of the following tests? What is the expected change in laboratory values as the pregnancy progresses?

   MSAFP: _____

   Estriol: _____

   hPL: _____

   L/S ratio: _____

8. M.W. is identified as being high-risk with her current pregnancy because her last pregnancy resulted in a fetal demise 2 years ago. She has been advised to check fetal activity daily at home. How will you instruct M.W. to use the Cardiff method to monitor fetal well-being? Include warning signs.

_____

_____

_____

9. J.C., who is 32 weeks pregnant, was involved in an automobile accident. You will be assessing her for fetal well-being. What are the advantages of external fetal monitoring for this client?

_____

_____

_____

10. S.L. is a 39-year-old, G2 P1, being seen for her first prenatal visit. She is concerned about possible genetic problems with this pregnancy because of her age and a family history of birth defects. What tests could be done to reassure S.L.? When could each test be done?

_____

_____

_____

11. Briefly describe the signs and symptoms and the medical–surgical management for the following obstetrical disorders.

	Signs/Symptoms	Medical–Surgical Management
Incompetent cervix		
Ectopic pregnancy		
Hydatidiform mole		

a. What follow-up care is important to the client with hydatidiform mole?

_____

_____

b. How would you explain the difference between placenta previa and abruptio placenta?

_____

_____

c. List several obstetrical disorders that can lead to DIC.

(1) _____   (5) _____

(2) _____   (6) _____

(3) _____   (7) _____

(4) _____

d. How can abruptio placenta lead to DIC?

_____

_____

e. What effect can each of the following disorders have on the fetus?

Maternal PKU: _____

Rubella: _____

CMV: _____

Herpes genitalis: _____

12. What clients are at risk of developing PIH?

_____

_____

_____

a. List the classic symptoms for PIH.

(1) _____

(2) _____

(3) _____

b. What are the three major goals of treatment for the client with PIH?

(1) _____

(2) _____

(3) _____

13. C.A., a 21-year-old primigravida, is diagnosed with PIH. Because her symptoms are mild at present, she can remain at home. What will you tell C.A. about home management for PIH?

_____

_____

_____

a. What factors might lead to hospitalization for C.A.?

_____

_____

14. M.A., a 23-year-old client, G1 P0, is O negative. Her husband is O positive. Will M.A. need RhoGAM during this pregnancy? If so, why?

_____

_____

_____

a. If this client is to receive RhoGAM, when would it be given?

_____

_____

_____

15. D.P. is a 24-year-old client with diabetes mellitus, type 1, diagnosed when she was a teenager. Her obstetric history includes two previous pregnancy losses, including a miscarriage last year. D.P. has poorly controlled diabetes as evidenced by high glucose levels and evidence of retinopathy. When asked, she admits she has not returned to her physician for diabetes management in "a long time." She is now approximately 10 weeks pregnant at her first prenatal visit. D.P. will be monitored closely for glucose levels and fetal well-being.

a. What effect will the pregnancy have on D.P.'s diabetes?

_____
_____
_____

b. In what ways might her diabetes affect the pregnancy?

_____
_____
_____

c. What are the risks for the fetus related to D.P.'s diabetes?

_____
_____
_____

d. D.P. tells you that she is very motivated to have a healthy baby with this pregnancy. What will she need to do to take care of herself while she is pregnant?

_____
_____
_____

e. How will the fetus be monitored during the pregnancy?

_____
_____
_____

f. How would preconception counseling have benefited D.P.?

_____
_____
_____

16. Fill in the table, which identifies high risk factors in pregnancy.

General	Obstetrical	Medical	Other

17. E.O., age 40, is a primipara and is at 16 weeks gestation. The obstetrician decided to recommend amniocentesis for E.O. Describe amniocentesis in terms that E.O. may understand.

    a. Describe how normal amniotic fluid looks.

    _____

    _____

    _____

    b. What laboratory tests are done on amniotic fluid? What are the tests for?

    _____

    _____

    _____

18. N.W. has been nauseated and vomiting into her second trimester of pregnancy. Why would the physician be concerned if N.W. were to become dehydrated?

    _____

    _____

    _____

    a. What types of medical treatment are indicated for hyperemesis gravidarum?

    _____

    _____

    _____

    b. What signs and symptoms could N.W. exhibit if she were dehydrated?

    _____

    _____

    _____

Self-Assessment Questions

Circle the letter that corresponds to the best answer.

1. You have been assigned to care for a client who is suspected of having HELLP syndrome as a result of PIH. You recall that this indicates your client may have all but which of the following complications?
    a. Hyperglycemia
    b. Lysing of red blood cells
    c. Decreased platelets
    d. Increased liver enzymes

2. The nurse is caring for a client with PIH who is receiving $MgSO_4$, a central nervous system depressant. To counteract respiratory depression that may occur with this medication, the nurse will be prepared to administer
   a. Narcan.
   b. Apresoline.
   c. epinephrine.
   d. calcium gluconate.

3. The nurse is caring for a client who is a 31-year-old multigravida diagnosed with gestational diabetes mellitus. Because of the effects of this disorder on the pregnancy, the nurse would anticipate a finding of
   a. macrosomia.
   b. hyporeflexia.
   c. oligohydramnios.
   d. peripheral edema.

4. The student is observing a fetal biophysical profile on her client, who is 35 weeks pregnant. The student recalls that this test should demonstrate fetal breathing and movement, fetal tone, amniotic fluid pockets, and
   a. a negative CST.
   b. a reactive NST.
   c. a negative Coombs' test.
   d. mild uterine contractions.

5. The nurse is caring for a client in active labor. The fetus is in a cephalic presentation at +2 station. With each contraction, the fetal heart rate is dropping after the acme of the contraction before returning to its baseline rate. The nurse determines that these are late decelerations caused by
   a. head compression.
   b. breech presentation.
   c. uteroplacental insufficiency.
   d. umbilical cord compression.

6. A nurse is performing an assessment on a client who is 33 weeks pregnant with a diagnosis of placenta previa. Which of the following findings will the nurse anticipate?
   a. Painless bleeding
   b. Abdominal rigidity
   c. Uterine tenderness
   d. Bright red bleeding

7. A general high-risk factor in pregnancy is that the client
   a. has diabetes.
   b. has had preeclampsia.
   c. has had a Cesarean birth.
   d. is unmarried.

8. The time of quickening is
   a. 8 to 12 weeks.
   b. 12 to 16 weeks.
   c. 16 to 20 weeks.
   d. 20 to 24 weeks.

9. When habitual abortions are caused by an incompetent cervix, it can be treated by
   a. a D&C.
   b. cerclage.
   c. a salpingectomy.
   d. induction of labor.

10. In an attempt to accelerate fetal lung maturity, a drug such as _____ may be given to the mother.
    a. betamethasone
    b. heparin
    c. methotrexate
    d. magnesium sulfate

The Birth Process

Chapter

3

Key Terms

Match the following terms with their correct definitions.

___ 1. Acme

___ 2. Amniotomy

___ 3. Augmentation of labor

___ 4. Bloody show

___ 5. Braxton-Hicks contractions

___ 6. Cephalopelvic disproportion

___ 7. Cervical dilation

___ 8. Cesarean birth

___ 9. Crowning

___10. Decrement

___11. Duration

___12. Dysfunctional labor

___13. Dystocia

___14. Effacement

a. Relationship of fetal body parts to one another, either flexion or extension.

b. Length of one contraction, from the beginning of the increment to the conclusion of the decrement.

c. Thin, fibrous membrane-covered space between skull bones.

d. Injection of a local anesthetic into the pudendal nerve to provide perineal, external genitalia, and lower vaginal anesthesia.

e. Condition in which the fetal head will not fit through the mother's pelvis.

f. Contractions that do not cause the cervix to dilate.

g. Unique ability of the muscle fibers of the uterus to remain shortened to a small degree after each contraction.

h. Labor with problems of the contractions or of maternal bearing down.

i. Expulsion of cervical secretions, blood-tinged mucus, and the mucous plug that blocked the cervix during pregnancy.

j. Relationship of the fetal presenting part to the ischial spines.

k. Relationship of the identified landmark on the presenting part to the four quadrants of the mother's pelvis.

l. Metal instruments used on the fetal head to provide traction or to provide a method of rotating the fetal head to an occiput-anterior position.

m. Condition of the umbilical cord being wrapped around the baby's neck.

n. Onset of regular contractions of the utuerus that cause cervical changes between 20 and 37 weeks' gestation.

___15. Engagement

___16. Episiotomy

___17. External version

___18. False labor

___19. Ferguson's reflex

___20. Fetal attitude

___21. Fetal lie

___22. Fetal position

___23. Fetal presentation

___24. Fontanelle

___25. Forceps

___26. Frequency

___27. Fundus

___28. Increment

___29. Induction of labor

___30. Intensity

___31. Interval

___32. Lightening

___33. Macrosomia

___34. Molding

___35. Nuchal cord

___36. Precipitate birth

___37. Precipitate labor

___38. Presenting part

o. Long, difficult, or abnormal labor caused by any of the four major variables (4 Ps) that affect labor.

p. Rotation of the fetal head back to be in normal alignment with the shoulders after delivery of the fetal head.

q. Incision in the perineum to facilitate passage of the baby.

r. Top of the uterus.

s. Medication that inhibits uterine contractions.

t. Peak of a contraction.

u. Stimulation of uterine contractions before contractions begin spontaneously for the purpose of birthing an infant.

v. Spontaneous, involuntary urge to bear down during labor.

w. Thinning of the cervix.

x. Artificial rupture of the membranes.

y. Irregular, intermittent contractions felt by the pregnant woman toward the end of pregnancy.

z. Manipulation of the fetus through the mother's abdomen to a presentation facilitating birth.

aa. Condition of the widest diameter of the fetal presenting part (head) entering the inlet to the true pelvis.

bb. Determined by the fetal lie and the part of the fetus that enters the pelvis first.

cc. Strength of the contraction at the acme.

dd. Enlargement of the cervical opening from 0 to 10 cm (complete dilation).

ee. Relationship of the cephalocaudal axis of the fetus to the cephalocaudal axis of the mother, either longitudinal or transverse.

ff. Increasing intensity of a contraction.

gg. Excessive fetal growth characterized by a fetus weighing more than 4,000 g (8.8 lb).

hh. Labor lasting less than 3 hours from the onset of contractions to the birth of the infant.

ii. Condition in which the umbilical cord lies below the presenting part of the fetus.

jj. Part of the fetus in contact with the cervix.

kk. Time from the beginning of one contraction to the beginning of the next contraction.

ll. Stimulation of uterine contractions after spontaneously beginning but having unsatisfactory progress of labor.

___39. Preterm birth

___40. Preterm labor

___41. Prolapsed cord

___42. Pudendal block

___43. Restitution

___44. Rupture of membranes

___45. Station

___46. Suture

___47. Tocolytic agent

___48. Uterine retraction

mm. Birth of an infant through an incision in the abdomen and uterus.

nn. Membranous area where sutures meet on the fetal skull.

oo. When the largest diameter of the fetal head is past the vulva.

pp. Resting period between two contractions.

qq. Decreasing intensity of a contraction.

rr. Descent of the fetus into the pelvis, causing the uterus to tip forward, relieving pressure on the diaphragm.

ss. Birth occurring suddenly and unexpectedly without a CNM/physician present to assist.

tt. Birth that takes place before the end of the 37th week of gestation.

uu. Shaping of the fetal head to adapt to the mother's pelvis during labor.

vv. Rupture of the amniotic sac.

Abbreviation Review

Write the meaning or definition of the following abbreviations and acronyms.

1. 4 Ps _____
2. AROM _____
3. CNM _____
4. CPD _____
5. FHR _____
6. LDRP _____
7. LMA _____
8. LMP _____
9. LMT _____
10. LOA _____
11. LOP _____
12. LOT _____
13. LSA _____
14. LSP _____
15. LST _____
16. PROM _____
17. RMA _____
18. RMP _____
19. RMT _____
20. ROA _____

21. ROM _____
22. ROP _____
23. ROT _____
24. RSA _____
25. RSP _____
26. RST _____
27. SROM _____
28. VBAC _____

Exercises and Activities

1. Briefly describe how each of these four variables affects labor.

   Passage: _____
   _____

   Passenger: _____
   _____

   Powers: _____
   _____

   Psyche: _____
   _____

   a. How do nursing interventions support the psyche of a client in labor?
   _____
   _____
   _____

   b. List six signs of impending labor.
   (1) _____   (4) _____
   (2) _____   (5) _____
   (3) _____   (6) _____

   c. How do contractions differ in true versus false labor?
   _____
   _____

   d. What are the expected changes for each of the following during labor?
   Temperature: _____
   Pulse: _____
   Respirations: _____
   Blood pressure: _____
   White blood cell count: _____
   Gastrointestinal (GI) system: _____

2. For the following diagram, identify the fetal presentation, lie, attitude, and position.

Draw an X over the place on the diagram where you would listen for the FHR.

Fetal presentation _____

Fetal lie _____

Fetal attitude _____

Fetal position _____

3. Complete the following statements.
   a. The first stage of labor ends when the _____.
   b. The delivery of the placenta occurs at the end of the _____ stage of labor.
   c. A client is pushing during the _____ stage of labor.
   d. Transition is part of the _____ stage of labor.
   e. The shortest stage of labor is the _____ stage.
   f. The second stage of labor ends with the _____.

4. On the following graph, draw in the labor pattern using the descriptions given.

   Frequency: 2 1/2 minutes

   Duration: 50 seconds

   Intensity: moderate

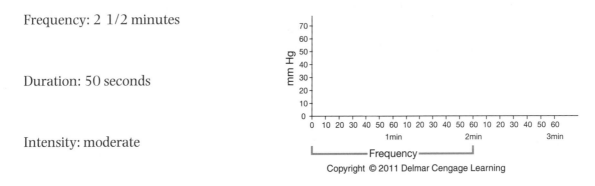

5. List two nursing interventions to support your client for each stage/phase of labor.

First stage:

Latent	1.	
	2.	
Active	1.	
	2.	
Transition	1.	
	2.	
Second stage	1.	
	2.	

6. Identify nursing interventions to support the mother and baby during the fourth stage of labor.

   _____

   _____

7. Using the following time lines, compare the length of each stage/phase of labor for the primigravida and the multigravida.

   Primigravida   5 hr   10 hr   15 hr   20 hr

   Multigravida   5 hr   10 hr   15 hr   20 hr

8. List risk factors for preterm labor.

   (1) _____

   (2) _____

   (3) _____

   (4) _____

   (5) _____

9. S.S. and J.S. have just arrived at the birthing unit for the delivery of their first child. S.S. is anxious and uncomfortable during her contractions. J.S. is excited about the birth and eager to help S.S. They attended all the childbirth classes but haven't been practicing the breathing and relaxation techniques. Describe nursing activities and interventions that can help S.S. and J.S. to feel welcome and comfortable during admission.

   _____

   _____

   _____

   a. List questions you could ask S.S. to obtain information about her labor.

   (1) _____

   (2) _____

   (3) _____

   (4) _____

   b. What information will be collected in the admission assessment?

   _____

   _____

   _____

   c. What effect can S.S.'s anxiety have on her labor?

   _____

   _____

d. S.S. needs support with her breathing techniques. How will you instruct S.S. and J.S. in the first technique?

_____

_____

e. S.S. had hoped for an unmedicated birth but is feeling overwhelmed with her contractions. A regional block is offered to her. List advantages and disadvantages of an epidural block for S.S.

Advantages	*Disadvantages*
_____	_____
_____	_____
_____	_____
_____	_____

10. Describe nursing actions for the immediate care of the newborn.

_____

_____

_____

_____

11. What are the five variables assessed with the Apgar score?

(1) _____   (4)_____

(2) _____   (5)_____

(3) _____

12. If the birth involves the use of forceps or is vacuum assisted, how might the infant be affected?

_____

_____

_____

13. How can you promote maternal/infant bonding after delivery?

_____

_____

_____

14. C.R., a 29-year-old, G3 P2, arrives on the birthing unit early in the morning with her husband. She tells you that she was awakened this morning with a contraction. She tells you that she had short labors with her last delivery. C.R. is full term and her pregnancy has been uneventful so far. Her membranes have ruptured. An assessment is completed and her physician has been notified.

a. Because C.R. is in the active phase of labor, how often will you check her vital signs, FHR, and contractions?

_____

_____

_____

b. If C.R. experiences a precipitate labor, what are the possible complications for her and the fetus?

_____

_____

c. C.R.'s labor is progressing well, but the FHR on the monitoring strip indicates that the fetal heart rate has dropped. C.R. is advised she may have a Cesarean delivery. List several indications for a Cesarean birth.

(1) _____

(2) _____

(3) _____

(4) _____

(5) _____

(6) _____

d. What preoperative procedures and support will be initiated for C.R.?

_____

_____

e. Following surgery with a horizontal uterine incision, the infant is suctioned, warmed, and assessed. Calculate the infant's Apgar score at 1 minute and 5 minutes.

	1 minute	*5 minutes*
Heart rate	96	126
Respiratory rate	Weak cry	Good cry
Muscle tone	Some flexion	Good flexion
Reflex irritability	Grimace	Crying
Color	Hands and feet blue	Body pink, extremities blue

Score

f. The next day, C.R. tells you she's just happy the baby is okay, but they had always hoped to have four children. Does this mean she has to have another Cesarean birth if she gets pregnant again?

_____

_____

_____

_____

_____

_____

15. What is the differxence between cephalic presentation and a breech presentation?

_____

_____

a. What are the three types of breech presentations?

_____

_____

16. What infection control practices do nurses use during labor and delivery?

_____

_____

17. B.K. is in active labor with her second child. She feels the need to push. As she begins to push, the nurse notes that the umbilical cord is protruding before head emerges. What actions should the nurse take immediately?

_____

_____

_____

Self-Assessment Questions

Circle the letter that corresponds to the best answer.

1. The fetus of a laboring client is noted to be macrosomic. The nurse realizes that this may predispose this client to a longer, more difficult labor known as
   a. dystocia.
   b. hypertonia.
   c. uterine inertia.
   d. dysfunctional labor.

2. The nurse is caring for a laboring client who will be having an amniotomy. The first nursing action following this procedure will be to
   a. test the fluid with nitrazine paper.
   b. assess the fetal heart rate for 1 minute.
   c. assess the mother's vital signs and level of comfort.
   d. perform a vaginal exam to determine the dilation and effacement.

3. A client in labor is using breathing techniques to deal with the discomfort. The client is using slow, deep chest breathing, which is no longer effective to deal with the pain of her contractions. The nurse will advise this client to
   a. take Demoral IM.
   b. try pant-blow breathing.
   c. use relaxation techniques.
   d. advance to shallow breathing.

4. A nurse caring for a client in labor identifies a prolapsed cord occurring with the spontaneous rupture of membranes. Which of the following positions will the nurse utilize with this client?
   a. Supine
   b. Lithotomy
   c. Modified Sims'
   d. Reverse Trendelenburg

5. The risks to the fetus in a breech delivery include all but which of the following?
   a. Fluid aspiration
   b. Precipitate birth
   c. Cord compression
   d. Head becoming stuck

6. The nurse is monitoring oxytocin augmentation with a client whose membranes have ruptured but who has exhibited poor labor progress. For this client, the goal for oxytocin administration is to promote
   a. cervical ripening.
   b. hypotonic uterine contractions.
   c. contractions every 2 to 3 minutes, 45 to 60 seconds in length, of moderate intensity.
   d. contractions lasting 90 seconds with a uterine resting tone of at least 20 mm Hg.

7. When is labor induced after membrane rupture with a near-term pregnancy?
   a. 6–12 hours
   b. 12–24 hours
   c. 24–36 hours
   d. 36–48 hours

8. The position that improves labor progression is
   a. prone.
   b. supine.
   c. side-lying.
   d. dorsal recumbent.

9. The client is alert and talkative and the cervix is dilated 3 cm. The client is in the _____ phase.
   a. latent
   b. active
   c. transition
   d. focusing

10. Which mechanism of labor generally occurs during the first stage?
    a. Internal rotation
    b. Expulsion
    c. Extension
    d. Flexion

Postpartum Care

Key Terms

Match the following terms with their correct definitions.

___ 1. Afterpains

___ 2. Attachment

___ 3. Bonding

___ 4. Claiming process

___ 5. Colostrum

___ 6. Disseminated intravascular coagulation

___ 7. Dyspareunia

___ 8. Engorgement

___ 9. Engrossment

___10. Entrainment

___11. Involution

___12. Let-down reflex

___13. Lochia

___14. Mastitis

a. Term for the first 6 weeks after the birth of an infant.

b. Neurohormonal reflex that causes milk to be expressed from the alveoli into the lactiferous ducts.

c. Incomplete return of the uterus to its prepregnant size and consistency.

d. Painful intercourse.

e. Long-term process that begins during pregnancy and intensifies during the postpartum period that establishes an enduring bond between parent and child and develops through reciprocal (parent to child and child to parent) behaviors.

f. Return of the reproductive organs, especially the uterus, to their prepregnancy size and condition.

g. Uterine/vaginal discharge after childbirth; initially bright red, then changing to a pink or pinkish brown, then to a yellowish white.

h. Newborn from birth to 28 days of life.

i. Discomfort caused by the contracting uterus after the infant's birth.

j. Infection following childbirth occurring between the birth and 6 weeks postpartum.

k. Formation of a clot due to an inflammation in the wall of the vessel.

l. Distention and swelling of the breasts in the first few days following delivery.

m. Abnormal stimulation of the clotting mechanism causing small clots throughout the vascular system and widespread bleeding internally, externally, or both.

n. Rapid process of attachment, parent to infant, that takes place during the sensitive period, the first 30 to 60 minutes after the birth.

____15. Metritis

____16. Neonate

____17. Oophoritis

____18. Postpartum blues

____19. Postpartum depression

____20. Postpartum hemorrhage

____21. Postpartum psychosis

____22. Puerperal (postpartum) infection

____23. Puerperium

____24. Salpingitis

____25. Subinvolution

____26. Thrombophlebitis

o. Inflammation of the fallopian tube.

p. Blood loss of more than 500 mL after the third stage of labor or 1,000 mL following a Cesarean birth.

q. Inflammation of the breast, generally during breast-feeding.

r. Condition more severe than postpartum depression and characterized by delusions and thoughts of self-harm or infant harm.

s. Process whereby a family identifies the infant's likeness to and differences from family members, and the infant's unique qualities.

t. Inflammation of the ovary.

u. Yellowish breast fluid rich in antibodies and high in protein.

v. Mild transient condition of emotional liability and crying for no apparent reason, which affects up to 80% of women who have just given birth and lasts about 2 weeks.

w. Parents' intense interest in and preoccupation with the newborn.

x. Inflammation of the uterus, including the endometrium and parametrium.

y. Infant's ability to move in rhythm to the parent's voice.

z. Condition similar to postpartum blues but which is more serious, intense, and persistent.

Abbreviation Review

Write the meaning or definition of the following abbreviations, acronyms, and symbols.

1. CNM _____
2. DIC _____
3. DVT _____
4. hCG _____
5. hPL _____
6. MSH _____
7. PPD _____
8. RhoGAM _____

Exercises and Activities

1. How do the parents and family members establish attachment with the infant?

_____

_____

_____

a. What behaviors by the infant are important in bonding and attachment?

_____

_____

_____

b. Describe nursing actions and interventions that can facilitate bonding.

_____

_____

c. J.B. expresses concern about how her 2-year-old daughter will react to the new baby. She does not feel they really prepared her for the birth. The daughter will be arriving with Dad in a little while. What guidance could you give J.B.?

_____

_____

_____

_____

_____

2. Briefly describe physiological changes that occur during the postpartum period in each of the following.

Uterus: _____

_____

Breasts: _____

_____

GI system: _____

_____

Urinary system: _____

_____

Musculoskeletal system: _____

_____

Blood values: _____

_____

a. What changes would the nurse anticipate in vital signs within the first 24 hours?

_____

_____

b. How do prolactin and oxytocin affect the postpartum client?

_____

_____

_____

c. R.L. tells you that she will not need to use birth control for quite a while because she plans to breastfeed her newborn son for a year. What information would you share with her?

_____

_____

3. What are the main tasks for the mother in each phase of maternal restoration and adaptation according to Rubin?

Taking-in phase: _____

_____

Taking-hold phase: _____

_____

Letting-go phase: _____

_____

a. List several nursing actions or interventions that can facilitate the taking-hold phase.

(1) _____

(2) _____

(3) _____

(4) _____

(5) _____

(6) _____

b. Identify what each letter represents in the acronym BUBBLE for postpartum assessment.

B _____

U _____

B _____

B _____

L _____

E _____

c. What other subjective and objective information is collected during the assessment?

_____

_____

d. List factors that cause discomfort in the postpartum client.

_____

_____

e. J.A. tells you during your assessment that she is having a lot of pain "in my bottom." What comfort measures can you offer or suggest?

_____

_____

_____

_____

4. How do postpartum blues differ from postpartum depression?

_____

_____

_____

   a. Describe why postpartum psychosis is a medical emergency.

_____

_____

5. Identify factors that predispose the postpartum client to infection.

_____

_____

   a. You are helping to discharge your client, T.Z., and her new baby today. The nurse asks you to review the signs and symptoms of postpartum infection with T.Z. before she goes home. What information will you include?

_____

_____

6. C.V. had a normal pregnancy and vaginally delivered a healthy girl. C.V. asks the nurse when she will get her figure back. Describe the process of involution in terms C.V. can understand.

_____

_____

_____

   a. C.V. asks when her vaginal discharge will end. Describe the changes that occur in the lochia.

_____

_____

_____

   b. C.V. also wants to know how soon her menses will resume. How should the nurse respond?

_____

_____

_____

7. D.P. is a 17-year-old single mother, G1 P1, who has delivered an apparently healthy baby girl 3 hours ago with a Cesarean birth. D.P.'s mother is with her in the room and is holding the baby. She smiles and tells you this is their second grandchild. There is no information about the father of the baby. You notice that your client is very tired and is dozing on and off.

   a. What additional assessment is necessary for D.P. because she had a Cesarean birth?

_____

_____

_____

b. What special concerns may be related to D.P.'s age?

_____

_____

_____

c. After D.P. has rested, you ask her if she would like to feed the baby. D.P. tells you that she would like to try to breastfeed, but she does not have any milk yet. What will you tell her?

_____

_____

_____

_____

d. The next day, D.P. has been encouraged to walk some and begin caring for herself and her baby. A few hours later, you notice D.P. is still lying in bed. She tells you she is too tired and too uncomfortable to get up. Why is it important for her to become more active? How can you help D.P. to balance her need for rest and activity?

_____

_____

_____

e. What observations might tell you whether D.P. is adapting to her new role as mother?

_____

_____

_____

_____

_____

_____

8. Describe the infection control practices that the nurse uses in postpartum care.

_____

_____

_____

9. Explain why Rh immune globulin is used following the birth.

_____

_____

10. Postpartum hemorrhage is a serious complication of childbirth. Identify causes of postpartum hemorrhage.

_____

_____

a. What medications may be given in the event of postpartum hemorrhage and why?

_____

_____

_____

Self-Assessment Questions

Circle the letter that corresponds to the best answer.

1. While assessing the postpartum client, the nurse makes the following findings. Which of these findings would *not* be expected during the first 24 hours after delivery?
    a. Diaphoresis
    b. Bradycardia
    c. Positive Homans' sign
    d. Temperature of 99.8°F

2. The nursing student is caring for a 39-year-old client who has given birth to her first baby. The student tells her instructor that the mother seems a little anxious and unsure of herself with her infant. She asks for help with infant care. The instructor reminds the student that this is
    a. typical behavior for an older mother.
    b. part of the taking-hold phase for the mother.
    c. a sign that the client is still in the taking-in phase.
    d. an indication of the mother's having a problem relating to her infant.

3. The nurse is assessing a postpartum client 2 days after delivery. The nurse notes that the fundus is firm, 2 cm below the umbilicus, she has lochia rubra with occasional small clots, and some edema of the perineum. The nurse will
    a. chart normal findings.
    b. medicate for uterine atony.
    c. note signs of puerperal infection.
    d. alert the CNM/physician to possible subinvolution.

4. The postpartum client is predisposed to urinary tract infection by all except which of the following factors?
    a. Urinary stasis after birth
    b. Trauma to the bladder and urethra
    c. Catheterization during labor or surgery
    d. Voiding every 2 hours after delivery

5. A new mother is breastfeeding her infant. At 3 days postpartum, she tells you her breasts are enlarged, warm, and tender. She also has a tingling or burning sensation in her nipples and a low-grade fever. The nurse advises the mother to
    a. use a breast pump to increase her comfort.
    b. discontinue breastfeeding and notify her CNM/physician.
    c. continue nursing the infant, because these are expected changes.
    d. supplement the infant with formula until her breasts return to normal size.

6. A behavior indicating that a toddler is adapting to a new infant in the home is:
    a. thumb sucking.
    b. bed wetting.
    c. hostility.
    d. independence.

7. The client's lochia is pinkish brown. This is called
   a. lochia rubra.
   b. lochia serosa.
   c. lochia alba.
   d. lochia drainage.

8. A laceration through the skin, mucous membrane, muscle, and rectal sphincter is considered
   _____ degree.
   a. first
   b. second
   c. third
   d. fourth

9. Oxytocin causes
   a. tingling and burning.
   b. milk expression.
   c. increased glucose levels.
   d. ovulation.

10. A mother who cares lovingly for her infant but is unable to feel love is experiencing _____
    postpartum depression.
    a. mild
    b. moderate
    c. severe
    d. transient

Newborn Care

Key Terms

Match the following terms with their correct definitions.

___ 1. Appropriate for gestational age

___ 2. Caput succedaneum

___ 3. Cephalhematoma

___ 4. Circumcision

___ 5. Cold stress

___ 6. Conduction

___ 7. Convection

___ 8. Cryptorchidism

___ 9. Down syndrome

___10. Epispadias

___11. Epstein's pearls

___12. Evaporation

___13. Foremilk

___14. Hallux varus

___15. Hindmilk

a. Maintenance of body temperature.

b. Whitish fluid secreted by a newborn's nipples.

c. Loss of heat when water is changed to a vapor.

d. Failure of one or both testes to descend.

e. Saclike protrusion along the vertebral column filled with cerebrospinal fluid, meninges, nerve roots, and spinal cord.

f. Production of heat.

g. Environment in which the newborn can maintain internal body temperature with minimal oxygen consumption and metabolism.

h. Infant's weight is above the 90th percentile for gestational age.

i. Metabolism of brown fat; process unique to the newborn.

j. Infant's weight falls below the 10th percentile for gestational age.

k. Small, whitish yellow epithelial cysts found on the hard palate.

l. Edema of the newborn's scalp that is present at birth, may cross suture lines, and is caused by head compression against the cervix.

m. Follows foremilk; is higher in fat content, leading to weight gain; and is more satisfying.

n. First few hours after birth wherein the newborn makes changes to and stabilizes respiratory and circulatory functions.

o. Collection of blood between the periosteum and the skull of a newborn; appears several hours to a day after birth, does not cross suture lines, and is caused by the rupturing of the periosteal bridging veins due to friction and pressure during labor and delivery.

___16. Hydrocele

p. Infant's weight falls between the 90th and 10th percentile for gestational age.

___17. Hyperbilirubinemia

q. Placement of the great toe farther from the other toes.

___18. Hypospadias

r. Inflammation of the newborn's eyes that results from passing through the birth canal when a gonorrheal or chlamydial infection is present.

___19. Kernicterus

s. Congenital deformity in which the foot and ankle are twisted inward and cannot be moved to a midline position; also known as club foot.

___20. Large for gestational age

t. Saclike protrusion along the vertebral column filled with cerebrospinal fluid and meninges.

___21. Meningocele

u. Loss of heat by direct contact with a cooler object

___22. Myelomeningocele

v. Fluid around the testes in the scrotum.

___23. Neonatal transition

w. Surgical removal of the prepuce (foreskin) that covers the glans penis.

___24. Neutral thermal environment

x. Placement of the urinary meatus on the underside of the penis.

___25. Nonshivering thermogenesis

y. Condition wherein the opening in the foreskin is so small that it cannot be pulled back over the glans.

___26. Ophthalmia neonatorum

z. Loss of heat by transfer to cooler near objects, but not through direct contact.

___27. Phimosis

aa. Excessive heat loss.

___28. Pseudomenstruation

bb. Failure of the vertebral arch to close.

___29. Radiation

cc. Blood-tinged mucous discharge from the vagina of a newborn, caused by the withdrawal of maternal hormones.

___30. Small for gestational age

dd. Watery first milk from the breast, high in lactose, like skim milk, and effective in quenching thirst.

___31. Spina bifida occulta

ee. Loss of heat by the movement of air.

___32. Syndactyly

ff. Excess of bilirubin in the blood.

___33. Talipes equinovarus

gg. Severe neurological damage resulting from a high level of bilirubin (jaundice).

___34. Thermogenesis

hh. Congenital chromosomal abnormality; also called trisomy 21.

___35. Thermoregulation

ii. Fusion of two or more fingers or toes.

___36. Witch's milk

jj. The placement of the urinary meatus on the top of the penis.

Key Terms Regarding Physical Characteristics of Newborns

___ 1. Acrocyanosis

___ 2. Erythema toxicum neonatorum

___ 3. Lanugo

___ 4. Meconium

___ 5. Milia

___ 6. Molding

___ 7. Mongolian spots

___ 8. Nevus flammeus

___ 9. Nevus vascularis

___10. Telangiectactic nevi

___11. Vernix caseosa

a. Shaping of the fetal head to adapt to the mother's pelvis during labor.

b. Large patches of bluish skin on the buttocks of dark-skinned infants.

c. Birthmark of enlarged superficial blood vessels, elevated and red in color.

d. Large purplish birthmark usually found on the face or neck that does not blanch with pressure.

e. Birthmarks of dilated capillaries that blanch with pressure; also called storkbites.

f. Pink rash with firm, yellow-white papules or pustules found on the chest, abdomen, back, and/or buttocks of a newborn.

g. White, pinhead-size distended sebaceous glands on cheeks, nose, and chin.

h. Blue coloring of hands and feet.

i. Fine, downy hair covering the fetus's body.

j. White, creamy substance covering a fetus's body.

k. First bowel movement of a newborn.

Abbreviation Review

Write the meaning or definition of the following abbreviations, acronyms, and symbols.

1. AAFP _____

2. AAP _____

3. ACIP _____

4. AGA _____

5. CPAP _____

6. FAS _____

7. HBIG _____

8. Hep B _____

9. IDM _____

10. ISAM _____

11. LGA _____

12. PKU _____

13. RDS _____

14. REM _____

15. SIDS _____

16. SGA _____

17. TTN _____

Exercises and Activities

1. List the four factors that help to initiate breathing in the newborn.

   (1) _____   (3) _____

   (2) _____   (4) _____

2. What four changes occur in the circulation of the newborn?

   _____

   _____

   _____

3. Describe how cold stress can lead to respiratory distress for the infant.

   _____

   _____

   _____

4. List the four methods of heat loss for the newborn and identify two interventions to prevent heat loss with each.

   (1) _____   (1) _____

                                            (2) _____

   (2) _____   (1) _____

                                            (2) _____

   (3) _____   (1) _____

                                            (2) _____

   (4) _____   (1) _____

                                            (2) _____

5. As a student nurse, this was your first birth. "Congratulations!" you tell J.M. and T.M. after assisting with the difficult but rewarding vaginal birth of a baby boy. They have already named him M., since they have known for some time it was going to be a boy. You are working today with Jan, an experienced labor and delivery nurse who enjoys working with students. Jan has already started taking care of M.'s immediate needs after birth, including:

   (1) _____   (3) _____   (5) _____

   (2) _____   (4) _____   (6) _____.

   Jan tells you, "We will be giving the baby an injection of vitamin K because:

   _____."

   "We also need to use erythromycin ointment because:

   _____."

a. You help Jan by assessing M.'s vital signs. They are, T—99.1°F; HR—154; R—62. Which are not in the normal range for vital signs? _____

b. Together, you and Jan have completed M.'s first physical assessment, noting all of the following findings. Circle those that could be due to the difficult delivery.

Acrocyanosis	Epstein's pearls	Edematous scrotum	Nevus vascularis
Cephalhematoma	Facial petechiae	Milia	Strabismus
Cryptorchidism	Flexed extremities	Molding	Subconjunctival hemorrhage
Ecchymosis	Lanugo	Mongolian spots	Telangiectatic nevi

c. J.M. says, "Why is his head shaped so funny? Will it stay like that?" What will you tell the parents about molding?

_____

_____

d. You check M.'s reflexes and demonstrate three of them for T.M. and J.M. Describe how to elicit each of these reflexes:

Palmar grasp: _____

_____

Babinski's reflex: _____

_____

Moro reflex: _____

_____

Draw a line under the reflexes that will normally be gone by M.'s 6-month checkup. Circle those that M. will need for breastfeeding.

Babinski's	Gallant	Placing	Sucking
Blinking	Hiccupping	Plantar grasp	Swallowing
Crossed extension	Moro	Rooting	Tonic neck
Extrusion	Palmar grasp	Stepping	Yawning

e. It is time to estimate M's gestational age. You will be using the New Ballard Score for this, which you have found in your text. Jan has already completed the neuromuscular maturity section for a score of 20. You offer to complete the physical maturity section. Draw an X on each block on the following scale that corresponds to the physical assessment findings.

He has some cracking on his skin, with rare veins.

Almost no lanugo remains.

Plantar creases cover the anterior two-thirds of the feet.

Breast tissue has a raised areola with a 4-mm bud.

The ears are formed and firm with instant recoil.

The testes are pendulous and have deep rugae.

	-1	0	1	2	3	4	5
Skin	sticky friable transparent	gelatinous red, translucent	smooth pink, visible veins	superficial peeling and or rash few veins	cracking pale areas rare veins	parchment deep cracking no vessels	feathery cracked wrinkled
Lanugo	none	sparse	abundant	thinning	bald areas	mostly bald	
Planiar Surface	heel-toe 40–50min: -1 <40min: -2	>50mm no crease	faint red marks	anterior transverse crease only	creases ant. 2/3	creases over entire sole	
Breast	imperceptible	barely imperceptible	flat areola no bud	stippled areola 1–2mm bud	raised areola 3–4mm bud	full areola 5–10mm bud	
Eye/Ear	lids fused loosely: -1 tightly: -2	lids open pinna flat stays folded	sl. curved pinna; soft slow recoil	well curved pinna; soft but ready recoil	formed and firm instant recoil	thick cartilage ear stiff	
Genitals Male	scrotum flat, smooth	scrotum empty faint rugae	testes in upper canal rare rugae	testes descending few rugae	testes down good rugae	testes pendulous deep rugae	
Genitals Female	clitoris prominant labia flat	prominant clitoris small labia minora	prominent clitoris enlarging minora	majora & minora equally prominent	majora large minora small	majora cover clitoris and minora	

Your total score for physical maturity is _____.
Added to Jan's neuromuscular maturity score of 20, this gives a total of_____.
Using the Maturity Rating scale in the text, what is his approximate gestational age based on this score? _____

Jan says that comparing his weight, length, and head circumference, M. is AGA. What does this mean?
_____
_____

f. Your instructor stops by and says you can give the baby his first bath. Why is a thorough cleansing of the infant important? How will you maintain M.'s temperature during the bath?
_____
_____
_____

g. You check on J.M. and the baby a few hours later. M. is quietly gazing into his mother's eyes and has very little body movement. He seems to be watching and listening to his mother intently. You realize that M. is exhibiting a behavioral state called _____.

h. J.M. and T.M. are considering circumcision for their baby. If M. is circumcised, what are your nursing responsibilities?
_____
_____
_____

i. During a final visit the next day, you find J.M., T.M., and M. together. J.M. is happy to see you because she needs some advice. The baby has been crying. J.M. says that a relative told her she ought to start feeding the baby formula instead of breast milk because he sounds hungry all the time. You remind J.M. that babies cry for other reasons, too, including:

_____

_____

You mention to J.M. some of the advantages of breastfeeding, including:

(1) _____ (5)_____

(2) _____ (6)_____

(3) _____ (7)_____

(4) _____ (8)_____

j. J.M. has a few more questions for you. Before you leave today, please go over them with her.

(1) "How often should M. breastfeed?"

(2) "How long should each feeding last?"

(3) "How can I tell if he is latched onto my breast properly?"

(4) "Since there is no 'air' in the breast, does M. need to be burped?"

(5) "How do I know if M. is getting enough milk?"

(6) "When do I take M. for his first doctor's appointment?"

_____

_____

_____

_____

_____

Self-Assessment Questions

Circle the letter that corresponds to the best answer.

1. A newborn has had difficulty maintaining its temperature within a normal range. The nurse recognizes that this can predispose the infant to
   a. cold stress.
   b. hyperglycemia.
   c. metabolic alkalosis.
   d. de-thermoregulation.

2. Which of the following physical assessment findings would the nurse observe in the preterm newborn with a gestational age of 35 weeks?
   a. Little or no lanugo
   b. Undescended testes
   c. Square window sign of 0°
   d. Creases on the anterior two-thirds of the sole

3. A nurse is caring for a new mother and infant. The nurse suspects transient tachypnea of the newborn because the infant is observed to have
   a. grade 0 on the Silverman-Anderson index.
   b. respiratory distress noted immediately after the birth.
   c. nasal flaring and a high respiratory rate several hours after birth.
   d. an irregular respiratory rate between 30 and 40 breaths per minute.

4. The nurse is caring for a new mother and infant after delivery. To facilitate mother–infant bonding and help initiate breastfeeding, the nurse will
   a. allow the infant to get hungry before beginning to breastfeed.
   b. leave the infant with its mother during the first period of reactivity.
   c. wait until the mother is fully rested after delivery to give her the infant.
   d. encourage mother–infant contact while the infant is in the active alert state.

5. The nursing instructor reminds the student to keep the newborn away from the cold window in the mother's room. This intervention will avoid heat loss in the newborn through
   a. radiation.
   b. convection.
   c. conduction.
   d. evaporation.

6. When an infant has nonshivering thermogenesis, it has:
   a. adequately raised its temperature.
   b. effectively increased its metabolism.
   c. now begun to metabolize brown fat.
   d. maintained heat retention.

7. A cold stethoscope is placed on an infant. The infant will have heat loss due to
   a. radiation.
   b. convection.
   c. conduction.
   d. evaporation.

8. A medication seldom used as an eye prophylaxis due to its lack of protection against chlamydial infection is:
   a. erythromycin.
   b. tetracycline.
   c. phytonadione.
   d. silver nitrate.

9. Bleeding from the cord is noted. The nurse should
   a. observe the cord bleeding for changes.
   b. check the clamp and apply a second clamp on the body side of the first one.
   c. clean the cord.
   d. check the clamp and apply a second clamp toward the outside of the first one.

10. Breast milk that has a higher fat content is called
    a. hindmilk.
    b. foremilk.
    c. colostrum.
    d. nutramigen.

Basics of Pediatric Care

Key Terms

Match the following terms with their correct definitions.

___ 1. Assent

___ 2. Child life specialist

___ 3. Emancipated minor

___ 4. Family-centered care

___ 5. Rooming-in

a. Health care professional with extensive knowledge of psychology and early childhood development.

b. Recognition that the family is the constant in a child's life, while the service systems and support personnel within those systems change (Shelton & Stepanek, 1994).

c. Voluntary agreement to participate in a research project or to accept treatment.

d. Practice of staying with the client 24 hours a day to provide care and comfort.

e. Child who has the legal competency of an adult because of circumstances involving marriage, divorce, parenting a child, living independently without parents, or enlistment in the armed services.

Abbreviation Review

Write the meaning or definition of the following abbreviations and acronyms.

1. BSA _____
2. DDST _____
3. EMLA _____
4. ID _____
5. IQ _____
6. NCHS _____
7. OBRA _____

Exercises and Activities

1. How does a child's developmental level affect the child's response to illness and health care?

   _____

   _____

2. Describe the nurse's role in supporting the child and caregivers. Why are prevention and teaching important aspects of this role?

_____

_____

_____

3. List three factors or interventions that can help the caregiver feel prepared for the hospitalization of a child.

    (1) _____

    (2) _____

    (3) _____

4. How does rooming-in benefit the hospitalized child and caregiver?

_____

_____

_____

5. Describe the role of a child life specialist in the health care setting.

_____

_____

_____

6. What measurements are assessed in the child under 2 years of age?

_____

_____

_____

7. What measurements are assessed in the child aged 2 years and older?

_____

_____

_____

8. Describe how to correctly assess the blood pressure of a child.

_____

_____

_____

9. Identify security measures used by health care agencies.

_____

_____

_____

10. You are caring for a young child who may need to have an extremity immobilized for several hours. What interventions might prevent the need for a restraint?

_____

_____

_____

11. If a restraint must be applied, what are your nursing responsibilities before and during its use? What documentation is needed?

_____

_____

_____

12. You are administering an oral medication to an infant. How would you proceed?

_____

_____

_____

13. During physical assessment of a child, several measurements are taken to ascertain normal growth and development.
    a. List the measurements in children under the age of 3.

    (1) _____

    (2) _____

    (3) _____

    (4) _____

    b. List the measurements for a child older than age 3.

    (1) _____

    (2) _____

14. You are caring for a 7-year-old child with a terminal illness. Identify two interventions that may be helpful for each of the following:

    The child: (1)_____

                        (2)_____

    Parents: (1)_____

                        (2)_____

    Siblings: (1)_____

                        (2)_____

    a. What support services might be helpful to the caregiver?

    _____

    _____

    b. How can the nurse deal with personal feelings of grief?

    _____

    _____

15. M. is the 3-year-old daughter of Y.T. and K.T. M. is scheduled to have heart surgery for the repair of an atrial septal defect (ASD) early next week. Other than concerns about the ASD, M. appears to be growing well and shows no developmental delays. She has not been hospitalized since birth. A quick recovery is anticipated.

    a. How can M. be prepared for the hospitalization and surgical experience?

    _____

    _____

b. Although Y.T. and K.T. have anticipated the surgery for some time, they are now anxious and have many questions. What resources can be offered or suggested to help them feel more comfortable with the experience?

_____

_____

c. What information will the nurse collect at the time of admission?

_____

_____

d. How can the caregivers be incorporated into the care of their daughter?

_____

_____

e. List specific safety measures that the nurse would incorporate for this toddler.

_____

_____

f. What are the advantages of discharging M. home as soon as possible after the surgery?

_____

_____

_____

_____

16. At what age may a nurse begin using a radial pulse in the measurement of vital signs?

_____

17. How does the nurse measure urinary output on a child in diapers?

_____

_____

18. Explain the procedure for instilling ear drops in a child.

_____

_____

_____

Self-Assessment Questions

Circle the letter that corresponds to the best answer.

1. The most important aspect for preparation of a child for hospitalization is
   a. preparation of the caregiver.
   b. completing a developmental assessment.
   c. assigning a child life specialist to the care team.
   d. using age-specific books and pamphlets with the child.

2. The nurse is preparing medication to be administered to a young child. The most reliable method for determining the amount of medication to be used will be based on the child's
    a. age.
    b. weight.
    c. body surface area.
    d. degree of symptoms.

3. A nursing student is assisting in a well-baby clinic in the community. It is apparent that further instruction is needed when the student
    a. assesses the pulse apically for 1 full minute.
    b. compares the head and chest circumference in a 1-year-old.
    c. measures the height in the 1½-year-old in a recumbent position.
    d. measures the chest circumference 1 fingerbreadth below the nipple line.

4. The primary benefit of anxiety reduction for the child who is facing surgery is to reduce the
    a. anxiety of the parents.
    b. blood loss during surgery.
    c. preoperative medication needed.
    d. frequency of vital sign assessments.

5. A child is scheduled to have the Denver II performed. The caregiver asks the nurse what the purpose of this test is. The nurse responds by saying that the Denver II is a measurement tool that will determine
    a. whether any developmental delays exist.
    b. the child's IQ.
    c. how well the caregiver interacts with the child.
    d. whether the child's height and weight are within norms.

6. Federal guidelines state that children over 7 years of age have the right to give
    a. conscription.
    b. assent.
    c. informed consent.
    d. enlistment.

7. Normal vital signs for a 3-year-old could be
    a. temperature 98.8°F, pulse 160, respiratory rate 40, blood pressure 65/30.
    b. temperature 97.5°F, pulse 130, respiratory rate 36, blood pressure 70/46.
    c. temperature 97.5°F, pulse 120, respiratory rate 20, blood pressure 76/50.
    d. temperature 97.5°F, pulse 110, respiratory rate 14, blood pressure 90/60.

8. Normal vital signs for a 1-year-old could be:
    a. temperature 98.8°F, pulse 160, respiratory rate 40, blood pressure 65/30.
    b. temperature 97.5°F, pulse 130, respiratory rate 36, blood pressure 70/46.
    c. temperature 97.5°F, pulse 120, respiratory rate 20, blood pressure 76/50.
    d. temperature 97.5°F, pulse 110, respiratory rate 14, blood pressure 90/60.

Infants with Special Needs: Birth to 12 Months

Key Terms

Match the following terms with their correct definitions.

___ 1. Abduction

a. Any intentional act of physical, emotional, or sexual abuse or neglect committed by a person responsible for the care of a child.

___ 2. Antipyretic

b. High-pitched, harsh sound heard on inspiration when the trachea or larynx is obstructed.

___ 3. Atresia

c. Surgical incision of the eardrum.

___ 4. Child abuse

d. Abnormal development.

___ 5. Circumoral cyanosis

e. Yellow discoloration of the skin, sclera, mucous membranes, and body fluids that occurs when the liver is unable to fully remove bilirubin from the blood.

___ 6. Colic

f. Lateral movement away from the body.

___ 7. Dislocation

g. Severe itching.

___ 8. Dysplasia

h. Displacement of a bone from its normal position in a joint.

___ 9. Erythematous

i. Impacted feces in the newborn, causing intestinal obstruction.

___ 10. Hypotonia

j. Large patches of bluish skin on the buttocks of dark-skinned infants.

___ 11. Intussusception

k. Forceful ejection (up to 3 feet) of the contents of the stomach.

___ 12. Jaundice

l. Lax muscle tone.

___ 13. Kernicterus

m. Saclike protrusion situated along the vertebral column and filled with spinal fluid, meninges, nerve roots, and spinal cord.

___ 14. Lecithin

n. Major component of surfactant.

___ 15. Meconium ileus

o. Telescoping of one part of the intestine into another.

___ 16. Meningitis

p. Drug used to reduce an abnormally high temperature.

___ 17. Milia

q. Characterized by reddishness of the skin.

___ 18. Mongolian spots

r. Condition of sudden, recurrent attacks of abdominal pain.

____19. Myelomeningocele

____20. Myringotomy

____21. Projectile vomiting

____22. Pruritus

____23. Stridor

s. Severe neurological damage resulting from a high level of bilirubin.

t. Absence or closure of a body orifice.

u. Bluish discoloration surrounding the mouth.

v. Pearly white cysts on the face.

w. Inflammation of the meninges.

Abbreviation Review

Write the meaning or definition of the following abbreviations and acronyms.

1. AGE _____

2. ASD _____

3. BPD _____

4. CF _____

5. CFTR _____

6. CP _____

7. CPAP _____

8. CSF _____

9. DDH _____

10. FTT _____

11. GER _____

12. LTB _____

13. NGT _____

14. PDA _____

15. RDS _____

16. RSV _____

17. SCA _____

18. SIDS _____

19. TOF _____

20. VSD _____

21. WIC _____

Exercises and Activities

1. Why is it important to understand the differences in the systems of the infant versus the adult?

_____

_____

_____

2. List differences in the respiratory tract of the infant that increase the risk for obstruction and aspiration.

_____

_____

_____

3. Describe the signs and symptoms of pneumonia that might be noted in the infant.

_____

_____

_____

4. List several nursing interventions for the infant with pneumonia.

(1) _____   (4) _____

(2) _____   (5) _____

(3) _____   (6) _____

5. Describe signs and symptoms of respiratory distress syndrome.

_____

_____

_____

6. How would you explain the cause of cystic fibrosis to the caregivers of an infant with this disorder? What symptoms would the infant or child experience?

_____

_____

_____

7. L. has just been diagnosed with her second ear infection in 3 months. What causes an infant to be susceptible to otitis media? What signs and symptoms should her caregivers watch for that would indicate an infection?

_____

_____

_____

8. What differences in the gastrointestinal (GI) system in infants increase their risk for GI disorders?

(1) _____   (5) _____

(2) _____   (6) _____

(3) _____   (7) _____

(4) _____

9. You are assessing for signs of dehydration in an infant with a GI disorder. What signs and symptoms would you note?

_____

_____

_____

10. How can fluid intake be encouraged in the infant who is at risk of dehydration?

    _____

    _____

    _____

11. W.'s caregiver tells you during her baby's 6-week checkup that he seems unusually colicky. She realizes that new babies cry a lot, but W. just cries for hours at a time. Nothing she does seems to help. What questions will you ask W.'s caregiver? What suggestions can you give that may alleviate his colic?

    _____

    _____

    _____

12. Z. is being assessed at the pediatric clinic 2 days after his birth for his first well-baby visit. A right-sided hip click was noted at birth. What other findings might indicate hip dislocation? What would treatment for Z. include?

    _____

    _____

    _____

13. What are signs of physical neglect and abuse in an infant?

    _____

    _____

    _____

14. List several safety measures that are appropriate for the child's first year of life.

    _____

    _____

    _____

    _____

15. You are caring for A., the new daughter of J.T. and C.T. A. is a full-term infant weighing 7 lb, 8 oz and is 19 in. in length. However, A. was born with a cleft lip on the left side and a cleft palate. Although C.T. and J.T. are thrilled to be parents, they are visibly distressed about this congenital defect. They wonder how she will eat, how they will care for her, and when her lip and mouth can be repaired.

    a. How will you support J.T. and C.T. following the birth of their infant?

    _____

    _____

    b. Why is an interdisciplinary approach important to A.'s care?

    _____

    _____

   c. Identify complications that A. is at risk for before her surgical repair.

_____

_____

   d. C.T. asks you to help her feed A. with a special bottle and nipple. What suggestions will you
       make to help with the feeding?

_____

_____

   e. When will the infant's cleft lip and palate be repaired?

_____

_____

   f. List nursing interventions that will promote healing following the repair of her cleft palate.

(1) _____ (4) _____

(2) _____ (5) _____

(3) _____ (6) _____

16. Complete the following table regarding cardiac anomolies by describing each element.

	VSD	ASD	PDA	TOF
Condition				
Blood flow pattern				
Manifestations				
Treatment				

17. The client has sickle-cell disease. Explain the signs and symptoms of this condition.

_____

_____

   a. Why is dehydration a serious problem for those with sickle-cell disease?

_____

_____

b. Identify the 5 As of managing sickle-cell crisis?

(1) _____

(2) _____

(3) _____

(4) _____

(5) _____

Self-Assessment Questions

Circle the letter that corresponds to the best answer.

1. The newborn who has a history of frank breech position, is large for gestational age, or is a twin is at greater risk for
   a. club foot.
   b. hypotonia.
   c. hip dysplasia.
   d. developmental delays.

2. A 10-month-old child is recovering from a sickle-cell crisis. To prevent a recurrence of a sickle-cell crisis for this child, the nurse encourages the caregiver to do all but which of the following?
   a. Delay immunizations.
   b. Avoid cold temperatures.
   c. Use prophylactic antibiotics.
   d. Maintain adequate hydration.

3. A 1-year-old has just experienced a febrile seizure. The nurse emphasizes to the caregiver that febrile seizures
   a. usually last for several minutes.
   b. do not cause neurological sequelae.
   c. increase the risk of seizure disorder in childhood.
   d. can be prevented by prompt administration of aspirin for fever.

4. When caring for an infant with acute gastroenteritis, it is most important for the nurse to assess the infant for
   a. dehydration.
   b. abdominal pain.
   c. intake and output.
   d. number of diarrheal stools.

5. An infant arrives at the community clinic with signs of an upper respiratory illness. The infant has mild stridor when active, a barking cough, and hoarseness. The temperature is 99.6°F, and there is a nasal discharge. It is most important to instruct the caregiver to
   a. increase fluid intake.
   b. maintain a humid environment.
   c. watch for signs of respiratory distress.
   d. suction the mouth and nose for mucus.

6. What is *not* considered a clinical manifestation of abuse?
   a. Bruises on the abdomen
   b. Multiple bone fractures at various stages of healing
   c. Withdrawal
   d. Mongolian spots

7. A clinical manifestation present in ventricular septal defect is
   a. delayed growth and development.
   b. dysrhythmias.
   c. increased respiratory infections.
   d. a machine-like murmur.

8. A clinical manifestation present in tetralogy of fallot is
   a. delayed growth and development.
   b. dysrhythmia.
   c. increased respiratory infection.
   d. a machine-like murmur.

Chapter

8

Common Problems: 1–18 Years

Key Terms

Match the following terms with their correct definitions.

___ 1. Acanthesis nigricans

___ 2. Comedone

___ 3. Encopresis

___ 4. Epistaxis

___ 5. Gowers' sign

___ 6. Rhinorrhea

a. Watery nasal discharge.

b. Passage of watery colonic contents around a hard fecal mass.

c. Whitehead or blackhead.

d. Hemorrhage of the nares or nostrils; also known as nosebleed.

e. Walking the hands up the legs to get from a sitting to a standing position (as in Duchenne muscular dystrophy).

f. A velvety hyperpigmented patch on the back of the neck, axilla, or antecubital area.

Abbreviation Review

Write the meaning or definition of the following abbreviations and acronyms.

1. AAP _____

2. ACIP _____

3. ADHD _____

4. ALL _____

5. APSGN _____

6. ASO _____

7. BMI _____

8. CPT _____

9. DMD _____

10. DTaP _____

11. ESR _____

12. FPG _____

13. HBV _____

14. HSV _____

15. IPV _____

16. ITP _____

17. JA _____

18. MCNS _____

19. MDI _____

20. MMR _____

21. OPV _____

22. PCOS _____

23. RAD _____

24. TIG _____

Exercises and Activities

1. What factors put children at greater risk for parasitic infections than adults?

   _____

   _____

   _____

2. How would you differentiate pharyngitis from influenza? Are there differences in the treatment?

   _____

   _____

   _____

3. What are early signs and symptoms of asthma? What assessment findings might be noted in children with chronic asthma?

   _____

   _____

   _____

4. J., a 6-year-old boy in your pediatric clinic, has been recently diagnosed with asthma. What information will you give to J.'s caregiver about ways to manage his asthma at home?

   _____

   _____

   _____

5. Describe the pharmacological treatment for asthma.

   _____

   _____

   _____

6. List signs and symptoms and the medical–nursing management for each of the following common pediatric disorders.

	Signs and Symptoms	Treatment
Impetigo		
Pediculosis		
Acne		

7. How would you detect scoliosis during a routine screening of adolescents?

_____

_____

_____

8. Describe symptoms that might be noted in a child with ADHD. What are the goals for nursing care for a child with ADHD?

_____

_____

_____

9. Identify several risk factors for suicide.

(1) _____ (5) _____

(2) _____ (6) _____

(3) _____ (7) _____

(4) _____ (8) _____

10. What behaviors might indicate to you that an individual is considering suicide?

_____

_____

_____

11. Of the following communicable diseases, underline those for which there is a vaccine. Circle those that are transmitted by way of respiratory droplets.

Chickenpox	Hepatitis B	Mumps	Roseola
Diphtheria	Measles	Pertussis	Rubella
Fifth disease	Mononucleosis	Poliomyelitis	Scarlet fever
			Tetanus

12. Identify four barriers to immunization.

(1) _____ (3) _____

(2) _____ (4) _____

13. The caregiver of a newborn tells you that she is concerned about having her baby immunized. She has heard that some immunizations can have serious side effects and cause long-term complications. What would you tell her?

_____

_____

_____

14. What is the nurse's responsibility related to immunizations and documentation?

_____

_____

_____

15. D., who is 9 years old, was brought in to the pediatric office by his caregiver. She tells you that he had a fever at home of 101°F, pain in his joints, and a pinkish rash. During the health history, his caregiver reveals that D. had an untreated upper respiratory infection with a bad sore throat about a month ago. He seemed to get over it at the time without too much trouble. D. is now suspected of having rheumatic fever.

a. List laboratory test results that might confirm this diagnosis.

_____

_____

b. What other signs and symptoms might D. exhibit with rheumatic fever?

_____

_____

c. Identify the goals of medical management.

(1) _____

(2) _____

(3) _____

d. What will D.'s treatment include?

_____

_____

_____

e. List long-term complications that can result from rheumatic fever.

_____

_____

_____

f. D.'s caregiver wants to know if he can ever get rheumatic fever again. What will you tell her?

_____

_____

_____

16. V., age 6, has tonsillitis again. Identify the symptoms of tonsillitis.

_____

_____

a. The surgeon performed a tonsillectomy and adenoidectomy. Describe this surgery in terms that V.'s caregiver might understand.

_____

_____

b. What actions should the nurse take when caring for V. in the postoperative phase?

_____

_____

c. Explain why the caregiver should avoid giving V. red or brown liquids immediately postoperatively.

_____

_____

17. Complete the following table regarding communicable diseases in children.

Disease	Transmission	Signs	Treatment
Chicken pox			
Diptheria			
Fifth disease			
Measles			
Mononucleosis			
Mumps			
Pertussis			
Roseola			
Rubella			

Self-Assessment Questions

Circle the letter that corresponds to the best answer for each question.

1. The nurse is caring for a child diagnosed with asthma. To reduce mucosal edema and improve the effect of a bronchodilator, the physician orders
   a. Alupent.
   b. Brethine.
   c. prednisone.
   d. theophylline.

2. Laboratory test results show that a young child has ITP. The nurse recalls that ITP is
   a. most common in school-aged children.
   b. cured with antibiotics if diagnosed early.
   c. a complication of a streptococcus infection.
   d. an autoimmune disorder that destroys platelets.

3. The nurse is performing an assessment on a child who is ill with rheumatic fever. All but which of the following findings might the nurse anticipate?
   a. Chorea
   b. Polyarthritis
   c. Strawberry tongue
   d. Subcutaneous nodules

4. A child with fever, headache, sore throat, and rash has just been diagnosed with scarlet fever. You explain to the caregiver that the child
   a. will be treated with penicillin.
   b. will have lifelong immunity after recovery.
   c. may have complications such as meningitis.
   d. is not contagious after symptoms have begun.

5. Home treatment for asthma may include all but which of the following interventions?
   a. Family education
   b. Chest physiotherapy
   c. Use of a peak flowmeter
   d. Restriction of physical activity

6. An elevated _____ is indicative of a recent streptococcal infection.
   a. ASO
   b. ESR
   c. C-reactive protein
   d. leukocyte

7. Mild hemophilia may
   a. be detected from bleeding from the umbilical cord.
   b. not be detected until a toddler becomes mobile.
   c. not ever show any clinical manifestations.
   d. be detected from bleeding from a circumcision site.

8. Itching around the anus may indicate which common intestinal parasite?
    a. Giardiasis
    b. Roundworm
    c. Pinworm
    d. Hookworm

Answer Key

Chapter 1 Prenatal Care

Key Terms

1. j
2. d
3. i
4. t
5. l
6. f
7. gg
8. aa
9. cc
10. m
11. z
12. c
13. tt
14. u
15. aaa
16. dd
17. fff
18. g
19. qq
20. bbb
21. v
22. ll
23. ccc
24. vv
25. yy
26. ee
27. xx
28. ss
29. uu
30. kk
31. mm
32. n
33. ggg
34. pp
35. rr
36. ddd
37. ww
38. eee
39. zz
40. hh
41. o
42. ii
43. hhh
44. p
45. y
46. a
47. r
48. w
49. b
50. bb
51. ff
52. jj
53. s
54. nn
55. e
56. h
57. oo
58. k
59. x
60. q

Abbreviation Review

1. American Society for Psychoprophylaxis in Obstetrics
2. Association of Women's Health, Obstetric, and Neonatal Nurses
3. bag of water
4. biparietal diameter
5. crown-heel
6. crown-rump
7. diethylstilbestrol
8. estimated date of birth
9. estimated date of delivery

10. gravid, para/term, preterm, abortions, living
11. glomerular filtration rate
12. human chorionic gonadotropin
13. Fetal hemoglobin
14. human placental lactogen
15. International Childbirth Education Association
16. last menstrual period
17. Nurses Association of the American College of Obstetricians and Gynecologists
18. over-the-counter
19. protein bound iodine

Self-Assessment Questions

1. a
2. d
3. c
4. b
5. d
6. a
7. a
8. d
9. b
10. d

Chapter 2 Complications of Pregnancy

Key Terms

1. d
2. l
3. e
4. c
5. h
6. m
7. a
8. k
9. n
10. f
11. r
12. p
13. s
14. u
15. b
16. i
17. o
18. w
19. g

20. q
21. t
22. v
23. j

Abbreviation Review

1. cytomegalovirus
2. contraction stress test
3. chorionic villi sampling
4. dilatation and curettage
5. disseminated intravascular coagulation
6. estimated date of birth
7. electronic fetal monitoring
8. fetal acoustic stimulation test
9. fetal biophysical profile
10. fetal heart rate
11. fetal heart tones
12. gestational diabetes mellitus
13. human chorionic gonadotrophin
14. hemolysis, elevated liver enzymes, low platelet count
15. human placental lactogen
16. herpes simplex virus type 2
17. intrauterine growth retardation
18. lecithin/sphingomyelin
19. magnesium sulfate
20. maternal serum alpha-fetoprotein
21. nonstress test
22. phosphatidyglycerol
23. pregnancy-induced hypertension
24. phenylketonuria
25. Rh immune globulin
26. small for gestational age
27. toxoplasmosis, rubella, cytomegalovirus, herpes virus type 2
28. vibroacoustic stimulation test

Self-Assessment Questions

1. a
2. d
3. a
4. b
5. c
6. a
7. d
8. c
9. b
10. a

Chapter 3 The Birth Process

Key Terms

1. t
2. x
3. ll
4. i
5. y
6. e
7. dd
8. mm
9. oo
10. qq
11. b
12. h
13. o
14. w
15. aa
16. q
17. z
18. f
19. v
20. a
21. ee
22. k
23. bb
24. nn
25. l
26. kk
27. r
28. ff
29. u
30. cc
31. pp
32. rr
33. gg
34. vv
35. m
36. ss
37. hh
38. jj
39. uu
40. n
41. ii
42. d
43. p
44. ww
45. j
46. c
47. s
48. g

Abbreviation Review

1. passage, passenger, powers, psyche
2. artificial rupture of membranes
3. certified nurse midwife
4. cephalopelvic disproportion
5. fetal heart rate
6. labor, delivery, recovery, postpartum
7. left mentum anterior
8. left mentum posterior
9. left mentum transverse
10. left occiput anterior
11. left occiput posterior
12. left occiput transverse
13. left sacrum anterior
14. left sacrum posterior
15. left sacrum transverse
16. premature rupture of membranes
17. right mentum anterior
18. right mentum posterior
19. right mentum transverse
20. right occiput anterior
21. rupture of membranes
22. right occiput posterior
23. right occiput transverse
24. right sacrum anterior
25. right sacrum posterior
26. right sacrum transverse
27. spontaneous rupture of membranes
28. vaginal birth after cesarean

Self-Assessment Questions

1. a
2. b
3. d
4. c
5. b
6. c
7. b
8. c
9. a
10. d

Chapter 4 Postpartum Care

Key Terms

1. i
2. e
3. n
4. s
5. u
6. m
7. d
8. l
9. w
10. y
11. f
12. b
13. g
14. q
15. x
16. h
17. t
18. v
19. z
20. p
21. r
22. j
23. a
24. o
25. c
26. k

Abbreviation Review

1. breasts, uterus, bladder, bowel, lochia, and episiotomy
2. certified nurse midwife
3. disseminated intravascular coagulation
4. deep vein thrombosis
5. human chorionic gonadotropin
6. human placental lactogen
7. melanocyte-stimulating hormone
8. postpartum depression
9. Rh immune globulin

Self-Assessment Questions

1. c
2. b
3. a
4. d
5. c
6. d
7. b
8. c
9. b
10. a

Chapter 5 Newborn Care

Key Terms

1. p
2. l
3. o
4. w
5. aa
6. u
7. ee
8. d
9. hh
10. jj
11. k
12. c
13. dd
14. q
15. m
16. v
17. ff
18. x
19. gg
20. h
21. t
22. e
23. n
24. g
25. i
26. r
27. y
28. cc
29. z
30. j
31. bb
32. ii
33. s
34. f
35. a
36. b

Key Terms Regarding Physical Characteristics of Newborns
1. h
2. f
3. i
4. k
5. g
6. a
7. b
8. d
9. c
10. e
11. j

Abbreviation Review
1. American Academy of Family Physicians
2. American Academy of Pediatrics
3. Advisory Committee on Immunization Practices
4. appropriate for gestational age
5. continuous positive airway pressure
6. fetal alcohol syndrome
7. hepatitis B immune globulin
8. hepatitis B
9. infant of diabetic mother
10. infant of substance abusing mother
11. large for gestational age
12. phenylketonuria
13. respiratory distress syndrome
14. rapid eye movement
15. sudden infant death syndrome
16. small for gestational age
17. transient tachypnea of the newborn

Self-Assessment Questions
1. a
2. b
3. c
4. b
5. a
6. c
7. c
8. d
9. b
10. a

Chapter 6 Basics of Pediatric Care

Key Terms
1. c
2. a
3. e
4. b
5. d

Abbreviation Review
1. body surface area
2. Denver Development Screening Test
3. eutectic (cream) mixture of local anesthetics
4. identification
5. intelligence quotient
6. National Center for Health Services
7. Omnibus Budget Reconciliation Act

Self-Assessment Questions
1. a
2. b
3. d
4. c
5. a
6. b
7. c
8. b

Chapter 7 Infants with Special Needs: Birth to 12 Months

Key Terms
1. f
2. p
3. t
4. a
5. u
6. r
7. h
8. d
9. q
10. l
11. o
12. e

13. s
14. n
15. i
16. w
17. v
18. j
19. m
20. c
21. k
22. g
23. b

Abbreviation Review
1. acute gastroenteritis
2. atrial septal defect
3. bronchopulmonary dysplasia
4. cystic fibrosis
5. cystic fibrosis transmembrane regulator
6. cerebral palsy
7. continuous positive airway pressure
8. cerebrospinal fluid
9. developmental dysplasia of the hip
10. failure to thrive
11. gastroesophageal reflux
12. laryngotracheobronchitis
13. nasogastric tube
14. patent ductus arteriosis
15. respiratory distress syndrome
16. respiratory syncytial virus
17. sickle-cell anemia
18. sudden infant death syndrome
19. tetralogy of Fallot
20. ventricular septal defect
21. Women, Infants, and Children

Self-Assessment Questions
1. c
2. a
3. b
4. a
5. c
6. d
7. c
8. a

Chapter 8 Common Problems: 1-18 Years

Key Terms
1. f
2. c
3. b
4. d
5. e
6. a

Abbreviation Review
1. American Academy of Pediatrics
2. Advisory Committee on Immunization Practices
3. attention deficit hyperactivity disorder
4. acute lymphocytic leukemia
5. acute poststreptococcal glomerulonephritis
6. antistreptolysin-O
7. body mass index
8. chest physiotherapy
9. Duchenne muscular dystrophy
10. diphtheria, tetanus, acellular pertussis
11. erythrocyte sedimentation rate
12. fasting plasma glucose
13. hepatitis B virus
14. herpes simplex virus
15. inactivated polio vaccine
16. idiopathic thrombocytopenic purpura
17. juvenile arthritis
18. minimal change nephrotic syndrome
19. metered-dose inhaler
20. measles, mumps, rubella
21. oral polio vaccine
22. polycystic ovarian syndrome
23. reactive airway disease
24. tetanus immune globulin

Self-Assessment Questions
1. c
2. d
3. c
4. a
5. d
6. a
7. b
8. c